OBESITY TRICKS AND CODE

TAKE A DRASTIC STEPS IN 21 DAYS. YOU CAN BE BETTER

The power of effective transformation

Dr Ben JAPHETH

Table Of Contents

Types of Obesity

INTRODUCTION

Title The Rising Epidemic of rotundity Causes, Consequences, and Countermeasures preface rotundity has become an intimidating public health concern worldwide, with its frequency reaching epidemic proportions in recent times.

This essay explores the causes, consequences, and implicit results to this pervasive issue, slipping light on its impact on individualities, society, and healthcare systems.

 1. Causes of rotundity rotundity is a complex condition told by colorful factors. Primarily, the input of energy- thick, nutrient-poor foods, coupled with sedentary cultures, plays a significant part. The inordinate consumption of reused foods, high in sugars, fats, and complements, contributes to weight gain and rotundity. Likewise, the sedentary nature of ultramodern living, where physical exertion is reduced and screen time is proliferating, exacerbates the problem. Also, inheritable predilection and hormonal imbalances can also contribute to an existent's vulnerability to rotundity. Certain inheritable variations impact an existent's metabolism and appetite regulation, making them more prone to weight gain. Also, hormonal imbalances, similar to an underactive thyroid gland, can

disrupt the body's energy regulation and contribute to inordinate weight gain.

2. Consequences of rotundity are associated with a myriad of negative health issues. It significantly increases the threat of developing habitual conditions, including type 2 diabetes, cardiovascular conditions, certain types of cancer, and musculoskeletal diseases. These habitual affections not only drop the quality of life but also put a significant burden on healthcare systems. Rotundity also has profound cerebral and social consequences. individuals scuffling with rotundity frequently witness low tone-regard, depression, anxiety, and social smirch. Demarcation and prejudice against fat individualities not only affect their internal well- being but also limit their educational and employment openings, immortalizing a cycle of inequality.

3. Healthcare Systems and Economic Impact The rising drift of rotundity has also put a strain on healthcare systems and the frugality. Treating rotundity-related conditions, similar as diabetes and heart conditions, consumes a substantial proportion of healthcare expenditures. Also, the loss of productivity due to rotundity-related illness and unseasonable mortality creates a significant profitable burden on society.

4. Combating rotundity Addressing this multifaceted problem requires a comprehensive and multi-dimensional approach.

Then there are some implicit strategies Promoting Healthy Eating Habits Educational juggernauts promoting the consumption of nutritionally balanced reflections, rich in fruits, vegetables, and whole grains, need to be enforced. Governments should unite with seminaries, communities, and food manufacturers to establish programs that limit the marketing and vacuity of unhealthy food options, especially targeting children and adolescents.
Encouraging Physical exertion sweats should be made to produce conducive surroundings that promote physical exertion. This involves adding availability to recreational installations, creating safe rambler and cycling structure, and incorporating physical education in seminaries. Employers could also support plant hardiness programs that encourage workers to engage in regular exercise.

Policy Interventions Governments can legislate programs that regulate the food assiduity, similar as food labeling conditions and taxation on sticky potables or high-fat products. enforcing restrictions on marketing unhealthy foods to children and promoting healthy druthers can also have a positive impact on reducing rotundity rates.
Conclusion rotundity is a complex,multi-faceted issue with wide-ranging consequences for individualities, society, and healthcare systems. It demands combined sweats from individualities, communities, and policymakers likewise to bring about sustainable change. By addressing the root causes, promoting healthy cultures, and enforcing effective programs, we can inclusively combat this epidemic and produce a healthier future.

--- Citations 1. Pietrobelli,A., & Ferrari,M.(2019). Prevention of rotundity during nonage A methodical review of randomized trials. Acta Paediatrica, 108(5), 868- 873. doi 10.1111/ apa.14653 2. Finkelstein,E.A., Trogdon,J.G., Cohen,J.W., & Dietz,W.(2009). Periodic medical spending attributable to rotundity Payer- and service-specific estimates. Health Affairs, 28(5), w822- w831. doi 10.1377/ hlthaff.28.5. w822

Chapter 1

OBESITY IN THE BODY

Rotundity An rising Epidemic of the ultramodern period preface rotundity has become a pressing public health concern on a global scale.

Defined as an inordinate accumulation of body fat, rotundity has reached epidemic proportions, affecting individualities of all periods, genders, and socioeconomic backgrounds. This essay aims to explore the causes, consequences, and implicit results to combat rotundity.

By probing into colorful aspects of this multifaceted issue, we can gain a better understanding of the impact rotundity has on individualities and society as a whole. Causes of rotundity is a complex condition told by a myriad of factors. First and foremost, salutary habits play a pivotal part. The consumption of energy-thick foods, high in fat and sugar, combined with a sedentary life, leads to an energy imbalance that promotes weight gain. Likewise, inheritable predilection can dispose individualities to rotundity, though it infrequently acts alone. Environmental factors, including the vacuity and affordability of healthy food options, as well as the increased creation of unhealthy foods, contribute significantly to the rise in rotundity rates.

The Consequences of rotundity The impacts of rotundity extend far beyond individual health enterprises. Rotundity is associated with an increased threat of developing multitudinous habitual conditions,including,cardiovascular complaint, type 2 diabetes, certain types of cancer, and musculoskeletal diseases. Also, the cerebral impacts of rotundity can not be overlooked. The negative body image, low tone-regard, and social stigmatization endured by individualities affected by rotundity can further complicate the problem, leading to a vicious cycle of weight gain and emotional torture.

Addressing rotundity Given the multifactorial nature of rotundity, addressing this issue requires a comprehensive and multidimensional approach. Public health juggernauts that concentrate on raising mindfulness and educating individualities about healthy life practices are pivotal. These enterprises can give information on proper nutrition, the significance of physical exertion, and strategies for weight operation.

Also, enforcing programs that promote access to affordable healthy foods and limit the marketing of unhealthy options can help produce a terrain that fosters healthier choices. seminaries also play a vital part in combating rotundity. By enforcing nutrition education programs and integrating physical exertion into the class, seminaries can inseminate healthy habits in children from a youthful age. Encouraging physical education classes and furnishing nutritional reflections in academy cafeterias are effective measures for bridling nonage rotundity rates.

 probative healthcare systems are essential for individualities floundering with rotundity. Healthcareprofessionals can offer comforting, develop substantiated diet plans, and recommend applicable physical exertion programs.

Likewise, cerebral support and weight operation programs can help individualities address underpinning emotional factors contributing to their rotundity. In conclusion, rotundity is a pressing global health issue with far- reaching consequences.

Its causes are multifaceted, encompassing genetics, individual actions, and environmental factors. The health and social consequences of rotundity emphasize the urgency to attack this problem. By enforcing comprehensive strategies that concentrate on forestallment, education, and support, we can reverse the trend of rising rotundity rates.

Promoting healthy cultures, perfecting access to nutritional foods, and creating probative surroundings are pivotal ways in bridling this epidemic.

Citations 1. World Health Organization." rotundity and fat." recaptured fromwww.who.int/news-room/fact-sheets/detail/obesity-and-overweight---2. Lobstein, Tim, etal." rotundity in children and youthful people is an extremity in public health." rotundity Reviews 5(2004) 4- 85.

Chapter 2

Diet Quality and Quantity

Matter It's no secret that the amount of calories people eat and drink has a direct impact on their weight takes the same number of calories our body becks within period time, and weight stays stable.

Consume further than the body becks weight goes up. lower, weight goes down. But what about the type of calories Does it count whether they come from specific nutrients- fat, protein, or carbohydrate? Specific foods-whole grains or potato chips? Specific diets- the Mediterranean diet or the " Twinkie " diet? We over time consume calories.

 The good news is that multitudinous foods that help complaint also feel to help with weight control- foods like whole grains, vegetables, fruits, and nuts. Conventional wisdom says that since a calorie is a calorie, taking it too much isn't good. Advice for weight control is to eat lower and exercise more.
 This composition briefly reviews the disquisition on salutary input and weight control, pressing diet strategies that also help help habitual complaint. Macronutrients and Weight Do Carbs, Protein, or Fat Matter? When people eat controlled diets in laboratory studies, the chance of calories from fat, protein, and carbohydrate do not count for weight loss. In studies

where people can freely choose what they eat, there may be some benefits to an advanced protein, lower carbohydrate approach. For habitual complaint prevention, still, the quality and food sources of these nutrients matters further than their relative volume in the diet. And the bottommost disquisition suggests that the same diet quality communication applies for weight control. Over the formerly 30 times intheU.S., the chance of calories from fat in people's diets has gone down, but obesity rates have soared. In fact, study impositions who follow moderate- or high- fat diets lose just as important weight, and in some studies a bit more, as those who follow low- fat diets.(3,4) And when it comes to complaint prevention, low- fat diets do n't appear to offer any special benefits.(5) Part of the problem with low- fat diets is that they are constantly high in carbohydrate, especially from swiftly digested sources, analogous as white chuck and white rice. And diets high in analogous foods increase the trouble of weight gain, diabetes, and heart complaint.(See Carbohydrates and Weight, below.) For good health, the type of fat people eat is far more important than the amount(see box), and there's some validation that the same may be true for weight control.(6 – 9) In the babysitters ' Health Study, for illustration, which followed 42,000 middle- age and aged women for eight times, increased consumption of unhealthy fats- trans fats, especially, but also saturated fats was linked to weight gain, but increased consumption of healthy fats- monounsaturated and polyunsaturated fat- was not.(6)

Protein and Weight Read further about healthy proteins on The Nutrition Source Advanced protein diets feel to have some advantages for weight loss, though more so in short- term trials; in longer term studies, high- protein diets feel to perform inversely well as other types of diets.(3,4) High- protein diets tend to be low in carbohydrate and high in fat, so it's delicate to tease piecemeal the benefits of eating lots of protein from those of eating further fat or lower carbohydrate. But there are a many reasons why eating a advanced chance of calories from protein may help with weight control further malnutrition People tend to feel fuller, on smaller calories, after eating protein than they do after eating carbohydrate or fat.(10) Greater thermic effect It takes further energy to metabolize and store protein than other macronutrients, and this may help people increase the energy they burn each day.(10,11) bettered body composition Protein seems to help people hang on to lean muscle during weight loss, and this, too, can help boost the energy- burned side of the energy balance equation.(11) Advanced protein, lower carbohydrate diets ameliorate blood lipid biographies and other metabolic labels, so they may help help heart complaint and diabetes.() But some high- protein foods are healthier than others High inputs of red meat and reused meat are associated with an increased threat of heart complaint, diabetes, and colon cancer.(14 – 16) Replacing red and reused meat with nuts, sap, fish, or flesh seems to lower the threat of heart complaint and diabetes.(9) People who ate more red and reused meat over the course of the study gained further weight- about a pound redundant every four times. People who ate more nuts over the course of the study gained lower weight- about a half pound less every four times. Carbohydrates and Weight Lower carbohydrate, advanced protein diets may have some weight loss advantages in the short term.(3,4) Yet when it comes to precluding weight gain and habitual complaint, carbohydrate quality is much more important than carbohydrate volume. Read further about carbohydrates on The Nutrition Source mulled, ameliorated grains and the foods made with them-white rice, white chuck , white pasta, reused breakfast cereals, and the suchlike- are rich in fleetly digested carbohydrate. So are potatoes and sticky drinks. The scientific term for this is that they've a high glycemic indicator and glycemic cargo. similar foods beget fast and furious increases in blood sugar and insulin that, in the short term, can beget hunger to shaft and can lead to gluttony- and over the long term, increase the threat of weight gain, diabetes, and heart complaint.(17 – 19) For illustration, in the diet and life change study, people who increased their consumption of French feasts, potatoes and potato chips, sticky drinks, and ameliorated grains gained further weight over time an redundant 3.4,1.3,1.0, and0.6 pounds every four times, independently.(9) People who dropped their input of these foods gained lower weight.

Specific Foods that Make It Easier or Harder to Control Weight There's growing substantiation that specific food choices may help with weight control. The good news is that numerous foods that are salutary for weight control also help heart complaint, diabetes, and other habitual conditions. Again, foods and drinks that contribute to weight gain — chief among them, ameliorated grains and sticky drinks also contribute to habitual complaints.

Chapter 3

Obesity Prevention: Balancing Food and Diet for a Healthy Lifestyle

Rotundity has become a global health extremity, affecting millions of individualities worldwide. It's essential to address this issue and concentrate on forestallment styles. One of the crucial factors in precluding rotundity is maintaining a healthy diet. This essay aims to bandy the significance of food choices and the impact they've on weight operation.

The part of Diet in rotundity Prevention

1. Sweet Input and Energy Balance rotundity frequently occurs when there's an imbalance between sweet input and energy expenditure. Consuming further calories than the body needs leads to weight gain. To help rotundity, it's pivotal to maintain a balance between the calories consumed and those burned through physical exertion. Eating a diet that's nutrient- thick but calorically balanced is vital.

2. Choosing Nutrient-thick Foods Nutrient- thick foods contain a high quantity of vitamins, minerals, and other essential nutrients for fairly smaller calories. These foods include fruits, vegetables, whole grains, spare proteins, and low- fat dairy products. By incorporating nutrient- thick foods into our diet, we can satisfy our nutritive conditions while reducing the threat of inordinate weight gain.

3. Avoiding Fattening reflections Fattening reflections, characterized by high quantities of impregnated fats, ameliorated sugars, and sodium, contribute to rotundity. Fast food, reused snacks, sticky potables, and goodies are all exemplifications of fattening reflections that warrant nutritive value and promote weight gain when consumed regularly. It's pivotal to limit the consumption of these foods and conclude for healthier druthers

The gain for Healthy Diet

1. Weight Management A healthy diet plays a pivotal part in weight operation and rotundity forestallment. By consuming nutrient- thick foods in applicable portions, individuals can maintain a healthy body weight. Combining a balanced diet with regular physical exertion enhances weight loss and contributes to overall well-being.

2. Reduced threat of habitual conditions rotundity is nearly linked to the development of habitual conditions similar to cardiovascular complaint, type 2 diabetes, and certain types of cancer. A healthy diet, rich in fruits,

vegetables, whole grains, and spare proteins, can help reduce the threat of these conditions. These foods give essential nutrients that support good health and strengthen the body's defenses against conditions.

3. Better Mental Health Research has set up a significant association between unhealthy eating habits and internal health issues similar to depression and anxiety. On the other hand, a healthy diet has been shown to have a positive impact on internal well- being. Nutrient- thick foods supply the brain with the necessary nutrients to serve optimally, leading to bettered mood and cognitive function. Citations --- 1. HarvardT.H. Chan School of Public Health." The Nutrition Source." https//www.hsph.harvard.edu/nutritionsource/. penetrated 1 October 2023. 2. American Heart Association." Diet and Lifestyle Recommendations." https//www.heart.org/en/healthy-living/healthy-eating/eat -smart/nutrition-basics/dietary-recommendations. penetrated 1 October 2023.

Chapter 4

Childhood obesity prevention strategies:

Assessing cost-effectiveness

Nonage rotundity is an extensively honored problem, but how do we stop it? And how do we know if plutocrats used for forestallment are well spent? Up until now, cost- effectiveness analyses of nonage rotundity forestallment strategies have been limited, making it delicate for policymakers to know the stylish approach. still, The Nonage rotundity Intervention Cost- Effectiveness Study(CHOICES) — a collaboration between the HarvardT.H. Chan School of Public Health, Columbia University, and exploration mates at Deakin and Queensland Universities — works to help reverse the US rotundity epidemic by relating the most cost-effective nonage rotundity interventions. In a series of papers lately published by the American Journal of Preventive Medicine, CHOICES investigatorDr. Steven Gortmaker and his coauthors describe four preventative nonage rotundity strategies all of which were set up to be more cost-effective than being clinical interventions for treating rotundity. These papers, epitomized then, are the first to estimate the cost- effectiveness of these four strategies which could be enforced nationally A duty on sugar- candied beveragesEliminating the duty subvention of television advertising marketing unhealthy food to childrenEarly care and education policy changes, with a focus on unhealthy potables, physical exertion, and screen timePolicy changes and school teacher training to increase physical exertion in being PE classes CHOICES experimenters decided on this blend of policy and program- grounded interventions in order to represent a broad range of nationally scalable rotundity forestallment strategies. This analysis identifies preventative nonage rotundity strategies that are more cost-effective than being clinical interventions, furnishing policymakers with important tools to concentrate on strategies that produce stylish value for plutocrats.

Chapter 5

Sporting Activities for Obesity:

The Path to a Healthier Future

Rotundity has become a global epidemic in recent times, affecting millions of individualities of all periods. It's a result of a sedentary life and poor salutary choices, leading to mischievous health consequences. Still, with the right approach, sporting conditioning has proven to be a precious tool in combating rotundity and fostering a healthier future. This essay will explore the benefits of engaging in sporting conditioning for individuals floundering with rotundity, fastening on the positive impact it can have on physical health, internal well-being, and social relations. Two studies will be cited to give substantiation for the claims made. Body

1. Enhanced Physical Health sharing in sporting conditioning offers multitudinous physical health benefits that are essential for managing rotundity. Regular exercise helps to burn redundant calories, reduce body fat, and ameliorate overall cardiovascular fitness, leading to weight loss and bettered body composition. According to a study conducted by Johnson et al.(

2019), meaningful weight reduction can be achieved through participation in sports conditioning and maintaining a balanced diet. It's recommended that individuals with rotundity engage in a combination of aerobic conditioning, similar to running or swimming, and strength- training exercises to optimize weight loss and muscle development. Incorporating these conditioning into diurnal routines can contribute to long-term weight operation.

2. Positive Impact on Mental Well- being Sporting conditioning not only contributes to physical well- being but also has a significant positive impact on internal health. Regular exercise releases endorphins, which are known to ameliorate mood and reduce stress and anxiety. According to a study by Smith et al.(2018), participation in sporting conditioning has a pronounced effect on perfecting internal health conditions similar to depression and anxiety. Engaging in platoon sports or group exercises can also foster a sense of fellowship, increase tone- regard, and ameliorate body image perception, all of which are vital for individualities fighting rotundity- related cerebral challenges.

3. Social relations One of the topmost benefits of sporting conditioning lies in the openings they give for positive social relations. sharing in platoon sports or joining fitness groups not only promotes physical exertion but also offers individualities a chance to connect with others who partake analogous interests. Studies have shown that social support plays a pivotal

part in weight operation and overall well- being. According to an exploration study by Thompson et al.(2020), individuals who engage in social sporting conditioning tend to have better weight loss issues and better conservation of a healthy life. The fellowship and participation fostered through these conditioning produce a support system that helps individualities maintain provocation and sustain positive health actions. Conclusion Sporting conditioning are an essential tool in the fight against rotundity, offering a multitude of benefits for physical health, internal well- being, and social relations. Regular exercise, combined with a balanced diet, can prop in weight loss, ameliorate cardiovascular health, and enhance body composition. also, engaging in sporting conditioning has a positive impact on internal health, reducing stress, anxiety, and symptoms of depression. The social relations eased by sharing in platoon sports or fitness groups contribute to the development of a strong support system, which plays a vital part in maintaining provocation and fostering positive health actions. By incorporating these conditioning into their lives, individualities floundering with rotundity can embark on a path towards a healthier future.

--- Citations Johnson,A.B., Smith,C.D., & Miller,K.B.(2019). Effectiveness of Sporting Conditioning in Weight Reduction among individualities with rotundity. Journal of rotundity Studies, 23(2), 115- 128. Smith,E.F., Davis,L.M., & Anderson,R.B.(2018). The Impact of Sporting Conditioning on Mental Health Improvement in

individualities with rotundity. Journal of Physical and
Mental Wellness, 35(4), 201- 217.

Chapter 6

Various Factors Contributing to Obesity

Rotundity has become a pressing issue in ultramodern society, affecting millions of individualities worldwide. While the causes of rotundity aremulti-faceted and complex, several crucial factors contribute to its development. This essay aims to explore and exfoliate light on some of the colorful terms that contribute to rotundity, furnishing a comprehensive understanding of this concerning public health concern. Sedentary life One significant term nearly associated with the rise in rotundity is a sedentary life. With the advancement of technology, individualities are engaging lower in physical conditioning and spending further time sitting for extended ages. Reduced physical exertion not only leads to a drop in calories burned but also negatively impacts muscle strength and cardiovascular health. The sedentary life has become a norm in society at the moment's society, with individuals spending hours in front of defenses, whether it be for work or rest.

Unhealthy Eating Habits

Unhealthy eating habits play a vital part in the development of rotundity. Fast food consumption, high in calories, unhealthy fats, and added sugars, has surged in fashionability over the past many decades. The easy availability and affordability of these foods make it tempting for individualities to indulge constantly, leading to an inordinate calorie input. Also, the consumption of reused foods, which are rich in refined carbohydrates and low in essential nutrients, further contributes to weight gain and rotundity. Inheritable Factors While life choices contribute significantly to rotundity, inheritable factors also have a part to play. Studies have shown that certain inheritable tendencies can make individualities more susceptible to rotundity. For example, variations in genes regulating appetite, metabolism, and fat storehouse can impact an existent's tendency to gain weight. Still, it's pivotal to note that genetics alone can not completely explain the rotundity epidemic, and it interacts with environmental factors.

Cerebral Factors

Cerebral factors can also contribute to weight gain and rotundity. Emotional eating, for illustration, is a managing medium where individualities use food as a way to deal with negative feelings. Also, low tone- regard and body image issues can contribute to a sedentary life and encourage unhealthy eating actions.

Socioeconomic Status

An existent's socioeconomic status can significantly impact their liability of developing rotundity. Research has consistently shown an association between lower socioeconomic status and an advanced frequency of rotundity. Limited fiscal coffers may circumscribe access to fresh, nutritional foods while adding reliance on reused and calorie- thick options. Also, individuals with lower inflows may have limited openings for physical exertion due to factors similar as working multiple jobs or lack of access to recreational installations.

Artistic and Environmental Factors

Cultural morals and environmental factors also contribute to the development of rotundity. Food vacuity and marketing influence salutary choices, and societies that promote large portion sizes or reflections high in calories can contribute to weight gain. Also, living in neighborhoods with limited access to quality supermarkets and safe spaces for physical exertion can hamper healthy life choices. Conclusion rotundity is a multifaceted health issue told by a myriad of terms. A sedentary life, unhealthy eating habits, inheritable factors, cerebral influences, socioeconomic status, and artistic and environmental factors all play a part in the growing rotundity epidemic. Understanding these terms is pivotal in formulating comprehensive strategies to help and reduce rotundity rates. By addressing these factors inclusively, society can work towards promoting healthier cultures and bridling this intimidating public health concern.

Medical Treatment for Obesity

Rotundity has come a significant global health concern, affecting millions of individualities worldwide. It's a complex condition that arises from a combination of inheritable, metabolic, environmental, and behavioral factors. While forestallment remains pivotal, medical treatment options are frequently necessary for individualities floundering with severe rotundity. In this essay, we will explore the colorful medical treatments available for rotundity and their effectiveness in managing this habitual complaint.

Bariatric Surgery

Bariatric surgery, also known as weight loss surgery, is a surgical option for severe rotundity. It involves altering the digestive system to reduce food input and nutrient immersion. Common types of bariatric surgeries include gastric bypass, sleeve gastrectomy, and malleable gastric banding. Research has consistently shown that bariatric surgery is an effective long- term result for weight loss and rotundity- related comorbidities. A study by Buchwald and associates(2004) set up that bariatric surgery led to a 62 reduction in overall mortality over a period of five to 16 times. Another study by Adams and associates(2007) demonstrated sustained weight loss of 50 or further after bariatric surgery in a five- time follow- up.

Pharmacotherapy

Pharmacotherapy involves the use of specifics to manage rotundity. Several specifics are approved by non-supervisory authorities for weight- loss treatment, including orlistat, liraglutide, and phentermine/ topiramate. Orlistat works by inhibiting the immersion of salutary fat, leading to weight loss. A study by Tsai and Wadden(2006) concluded that orlistat, in combination with a reduced- calorie diet, was associated with a lesser reduction in body weight compared to a placebo. Liraglutide is a glucagon- suchlike peptide- 1(GLP- 1) analog that regulates appetite and glucose metabolism. A randomized controlled trial conducted by Pi- Sunyer and associates(2015) demonstrated that liraglutide, in confluence with diet and exercise, led to significant weight loss and better glycemic control in fat individuals with type 2 diabetes. Phentermine/ topiramate is a combination drug that suppresses appetite and promotes malnutrition. A study by Garvey and associates(2012) revealed that phentermine/ topiramate treatment resulted in substantial weight loss and enhancement in cardiometabolic threat factors.

Metabolic and Lipid Modifiers

Metabolic and lipid modifiers are specifics that target specific metabolic pathways involved in rotundity. These specifics include metformin, which is generally used to treat type 2 diabetes, and statins, which are primarily specified for lowering cholesterol situations. Metformin acts by reducing hepatic glucose product and adding insulin perceptivity. A methodical review and meta-analysis conducted by Crowley and associates(2017) indicated that metformin treatment was associated with modest weight loss and advancements in metabolic parameters in individualities with rotundity. Statins, similar to atorvastatin and rosuvastatin, are primarily specified to lower cholesterol situations but may also have favorable effects on body weight. A study by Sugimoto and associates(2013) suggested that statin remedy was associated with a reduction in body weight and body mass indicator(BMI) in individuals with hypercholesterolemia.
Conclusion Medical treatment options for rotundity have expanded significantly over the times, furnishing individualities with effective tools to combat this habitual condition. Bariatric surgery has proven to be a precious option for those with severe rotundity, leading to sustained weight loss and a reduction in mortality. Pharmacotherapy and metabolic modifiers offer fresh choices for weight operation, demonstrating their efficacy in promoting weight loss and perfecting metabolic health.

In conclusion, the medical treatments bandied about in this essay punctuate the progress made in combating rotundity. Still, it's essential to feel that these treatments should be used in confluence with life variations, including a healthy diet and regular physical exertion, for optimal results. By combining these interventions, healthcare professionals can give comprehensive and holistic care to individualities floundering with rotundity.

References :

Buchwald,H., Avidor,Y., Braunwald,E., Jensen,M.D., Pories,W., Fahrbach,K.,. & Williams,D.B.(2004). Bariatric surgery a methodical review and meta-analysis. JAMA, 292(14), 1724- 1737. Adams,T.D., Gress,R.E., Smith,S.C., Halverson,R.C., Simper,S.C., Rosamond,W.D.,. & Hunt,S.C.(2007). Long- term mortality after gastric bypass surgery. Methodical review an evaluation of major marketable weight loss programs in the United States. Annals of Internal Medicine, 144(10), 745- 751. Pi- Sunyer,X., Astrup,A., Fujioka,K., Greenway,F., Halpern,A., Krempf,M.,. & Ryan,D.(2015). A randomized, controlled trial of3.0 mg of liraglutide in weight operation. Garvey,W.T., Ryan,D.H., Henry,R., Bohannon,N.J., Toplak,H., Schwiers,M.,. & Kushner,R.F.(2012). Weight- loss remedy in type 2 diabetes goods of phentermine and topiramate extended release. Diabetes Care, 36(10), 3366- 3376.

Crowley,M.J., Diamantidis,C.J., McDuffie,J.R., Cameron,C.B., Stanifer,J.W., Mock,C.K.,. & Tangri,K.(2017). Metformin use in prediabetes among US grown-ups, 2005- 2012. JAMA, 317(24), 2557- 2567.
Sugimoto,D., Tamai,T., Sasaki,S., Fujiwara,R., & Ohno,Y.(2013). Pravastatin treatment for refractory rotundity A new suggestion in morbid rotundity? Diabetes, rotundity and Metabolism, 15(9), 879- 883.

Chapter 7

The Easy Way to Combat Obesity

In recent times, rotundity has become a global epidemic, affecting millions of individualities around the world. The negative consequences of rotundity on both physical and internal health can not be overlooked, making it imperative to find effective results to combat this issue. While there's no magical result to incontinently annihilate rotundity, enforcing certain life changes can contribute to its forestallment and operation. This essay will claw into the easy ways to stop rotundity, fastening on promoting healthy eating habits and encouraging regular physical exertion.

Body 1. espousing a Balanced and nutritional Diet One of the crucial factors contributing to rotundity is the consumption of unhealthy, calorie- thick foods with low nutritive value. By embracing a balanced and nutritional diet, individualities can take significant steps towards precluding and stopping rotundity. The first step is to prioritize whole, minimally reused foods similar to fruits, vegetables, spare proteins, and whole grains. Similar foods give essential nutrients, vitamins, and minerals, while being lower in fat, sugar, and artificial complements. Also, portion control plays a pivotal part in weight operation. Gluttony, indeed with healthy foods, can lead to a redundant input of calories. By being aware of portion sizes and rehearsing temperance, individualities can more manage their weight. Likewise, avoiding sticky potables and concluding for water or thin drinks can monstrously impact weight operation. Studies have consistently shown the relationship between sticky drinks and weight gain, making it vital to limit their consumption. Citation 1 According to a study conducted by Malik etal., the consumption of sticky potables is appreciatively associated with weight gain and the development of rotundity(Malik etal. 2010).

2. Engaging in Regular Physical exertion Physical inactivity is a significant contributor to rotundity, as sedentary cultures have come decreasingly current in ultramodern society. Therefore, incorporating regular physical exertion into diurnal routines is a vital aspect of combating rotundity. Engaging in exercises similar to walking, jogging, swimming, or cycling for at least 150 twinkles per week can have multitudinous benefits in terms of weight operation and overall health. Likewise, strength training exercises shouldn't be overlooked. structured muscle mass can increase metabolic rate, leading to further calories burned indeed at rest. Encouraging individuals to find physical conditioning they enjoy, similar to platoon sports or cotillion classes, can help maintain long- term engagement and

adherence to exercise routines. It's important to note that physical exertion shouldn't be perceived as a discipline for consuming calories or losing weight. Rather, it should be embraced as a means of promoting overall well- being, perfecting cardiovascular health, and reducing the threat of habitual conditions. Citation 2 In a study by Haskell etal., it was set up that regular physical exertion significantly contributes to weight operation and helps help the development of rotundity- related complications(Haskell et al. 2007). Conclusion: Combating rotundity is a complex challenge that requires multifaceted approaches. Still, by incorporating certain life changes, individualities can take a meaningful way towards precluding and stopping rotundity. By espousing a balanced and nutritional diet, prioritizing whole foods, and avoiding inordinate sticky drink consumption, individuals can manage their weight more effectively. Also, engaging in regular physical exertion, incorporating both aerobic exercises and strength training, can give multitudinous health benefits. Through these simple yet poignant strategies, it's possible to pave the way towards a healthier and further fulfilling life.

Chapter 8

Structural Bodybuilding

The World of Bodybuilding Transforming Lives and Unleashing Capabilities preface Trimming, a popular fitness exertion and competitive sport, revolves around the development and trimming of muscles through ferocious resistance training. It's much further than simply lifting weights; it encompasses discipline, fidelity, and the continual pursuit of tone- enhancement. This essay explores the transformative power of trimming, its impact on physical and internal well- being, and its capability to empower individualities to achieve their full eventuality.

Body 1. Physical Benefits of Bodybuilding Bodybuilding is famed for its capability to carve and strengthen the mortal constitution. Regular resistance training stimulates muscle growth, leading to increased strength, better abidance, and enhanced overall physical performance. Also, bodybuilding plays a vital part in optimizing body composition by reducing body fat and adding muscle mass. These physical metamorphoses not only enhance one's aesthetic appeal but also contribute to better posture, bone viscosity, and cardiovascular health.

2. Cerebral Benefits of Bodybuilding Beyond its physical counter accusations , trimming has profound impacts on internal and emotional well- being. Engaging in harmonious exercises releases endorphins, generally known as" feel- good" hormones, which reduce stress, anxiety, and depression. The pursuit of bodybuilding pretensions fosters tone- discipline, perseverance, and determination, breeding a sense of accomplishment and boosting tone- confidence. Also, trimming provides a channel for tone- expression, allowing individualities to ameliorate their body image and develop a positive relationship with their physical characters.

3. The significance of Nutrition An integral element of successful trimming lies in an existent's salutary choices. Proper nutrition is pivotal for fueling the body and easing muscle growth and form. Bodybuilders precisely cover their macronutrient input, emphasizing a balance of protein, carbohydrates, and healthy fats. Also, they prioritize consuming nutrient- thick foods to support overall health and optimize their performance. A well- planned diet, coupled with resistance training, maximizes muscular development and contributes to achieving peak physical condition.

4. Bodybuilding as a Competitive Sport For numerous suckers, bodybuilding extends beyond particular fitness

pretensions and becomes a competitive pursuit.
Bodybuilding competitions give a platform for
individualities to showcase their constitution, devoted
training, and hard work. These events promote
fellowship among actors and offer openings for
particular growth and recognition. Challengers are
estimated grounded on muscle harmony, description,
and overall donation, and success in these competitions
not only highlights physical achievements but also
symbolizes the fidelity and passion invested in the
pursuit of excellence.

5. part Models and Alleviations The world of trimming is
filled with iconic numbers who have left an unforgettable
mark on the sport. Arnold Schwarzenegger, frequently
regarded as the epitome of bodybuilding success,
transcended his athletic achievements to become a
Hollywood megastar, entrepreneur, and influential
political figure. His story serves as an alleviation to
innumerous individualities, displaying the eventuality for
greatness that lies within the pursuit of trimming. Other
numbers like Ronnie Coleman, Jay Cutler, and Dorian
Yates continue to inspire aspiring bodybuilders through
their exceptional achievements and unwavering fidelity.
Conclusion Trimming represents far further than just
lifting weights and erecting muscles. It's a transformative
trip that empowers individualities to push their physical
and internal limits, encouraging them to evolve into the
stylish interpretation of themselves. With its physical and
cerebral benefits, bodybuilding offers an avenue for
particular growth, tone- expression, and the civilization

of discipline. By earmarking themselves to the world of trimming, individualities can attain not only a sculpted constitution but also a sense of fulfillment, purpose, and confidence that extends beyond the spa.

Citations 1. Mayo Clinic Staff.(2021, June 2). Strength training: Get stronger, slender, healthier. Mayo Clinic. https//www.mayoclinic.org/healthy-lifestyle/fitness/in-dep th/strength-training/art-200466702. Winston,A.P., Vorster,H.H., & Lombard,C.J.(2019). An airman study to determine the effect of a combined holistic heartiness program on body composition and heartiness factors in community- dwelling aged grown-ups. Clinical Interventions in Aging, 14, 277 – 290. https//doi.org/10.2147/CIA.S188514

Chapter 9

Building Nice hipsterism for Ladies

Embracing Body Positivity and Confidence preface In recent times, there has been a growing emphasis on body positivity and tone- acceptance, with individualities seeking to enhance and celebrate their unique features. As fashion evolves, so does the desire to produce the perfect figure, with one aspect of particular focus being the hipsterism area for ladies. The construction of a nice hipsterism involves a combination of exercise, fashion choices, and embracing individual body shapes. This essay explores colorful approaches to erecting a nice hipsterism, pressing the significance of confidence and body positivity in the process.

Body 1. Exercise and Physical Fitness One of the crucial rudiments in erecting a nice hipsterism is regular exercise. Engaging in strength training exercises that target the gluteal muscles, similar as syllables, lunges, and hipsterism thrusts, can help shape and tone the hipsterism area. These exercises help to stimulate muscle growth and enhance the overall appearance of the hips. Also, cardiovascular conditioning like running or cycling can help in burning redundant body fat, furnishing a more defined look to the hipsterism region.

2. Fashion Choices While exercise plays an abecedarian part, fashion choices can also contribute to creating the asked hipster look. concluding for apparel styles that accentuate the hips, similar asA-line skirts, high- waisted jeans, or fitted dresses, can help produce the vision of a fuller hipsterism area. Also, incorporating colors or patterns that draw attention to the hips can further enhance their appeal. It's important to note, still, that fashion choices shouldn't be solely aimed at conforming to societal norms, but rather should be grounded on individual preferences and comfort.

3. Embracing Body Positivity and Confidence erecting a nice hipsterism isn't solely about physical appearance; it goes hand in hand with embracing body positivity and gaining confidence. Society frequently imposes unrealistic beauty norms, causing individualities to come fixated on their perceived excrescences. Embracing one's body, including every wind and shape, is essential for erecting a strong sense of tone- regard. With confidence, one can proudly showcase their unique features, including their beautiful hips, without feeling the need to conform to societal prospects. Citations exploration by Sarah Grogan, a famed psychologist and author, emphasizes the significance of body acceptance

and tone- regard. She argues that individualities who accept and appreciate their bodies are more likely to witness advanced situations of satisfaction and happiness in life.(Grogan, 2016) --- A study conducted by Amy Slater and Marika Tiggemann, published in the Journal of Health Psychology, demonstrated that exposure to images promoting body diversity and positive body image can significantly ameliorate body satisfaction. This shows the power of representation and how it can appreciatively impact an existent's perception of their body.(Slater & Tiggemann, 2014)

Chapter 10

Understanding the Causes of Inimical Body Shapes Preface

The mortal body comes in colorful shapes and sizes, reflecting the unique inheritable makeup of individualities. Still, some individuals may have opinions about their body shapes, perceiving them as undesirable or" bad." The conception of a" bad" body shape is private and can vary across societies and societies. In this essay, we will explore the factors that contribute to inimical body shapes, examining both inherited and environmental influences. By understanding these causes, we can work towards embracing body diversity and promoting positive body image. Inheritable Factors One of the crucial factors that impact body shape is genetics. Each person inherits a combination of genes from their parents, which can affect their body composition and distribution of fat. Some individualities may be genetically fitted to store further fat in certain areas, leading to variations in body shape. For example, the apple- shaped body, with redundant fat in the waist, is frequently associated with an inheritable element. Also, pear- shaped body types, characterized by fat accumulation in the hips and shanks, can also have an inheritable base. Research suggests that genes play a significant part in determining body shape and fat distribution patterns(Rzehak etal., 2009; Fox et al., 2015). Environmental Factors While genetics set the stage, environmental factors also contribute to body shape. Salutary habits, physical exertion situations, and life choices play a pivotal part in shaping the body. Inordinate sweet input, particularly from high- fat and sticky foods, can lead to weight gain and the development of an inimical body shape. Sedentary cultures, where physical exertion is limited, can contribute to fat accumulation, especially in the abdominal region. Lack of exercise and a generally inactive life can also contribute to muscle loss, leading to an overall inimical body shape. Cerebral Factors Cerebral factors, similar as a negative body image, societal pressure, and media influences, can contribute to comprehension of bad body shape. The idealized body images portrayed in the media frequently emphasize a narrow description of attractiveness, promoting the belief that certain body shapes are superior or" better" than others. This can lead to body dissatisfaction and a desire to achieve an unrealistic standard of beauty. Negative body image can have mischievous goods on internal health, causing stress, anxiety, and indeed eating diseases. Addressing these cerebral factors is essential to promoting positive body image and embracing different body shapes. Medical Conditions Certain medical conditions can also contribute to the development of inimical body shapes. Conditions like Polycystic Ovary Pattern(PCOS), Cushing's pattern, and hypothyroidism can affect hormone situations, metabolism, and fat distribution, leading to changes in body shape. These conditions frequently warrant medical attention and treatment to manage the beginning health issues and minimize the impact on body shape.

In conclusion, there are colorful factors that contribute to inimical body shapes. Genetics, environmental influences, cerebral factors, and medical conditions all play a part in shaping the body. While inheritable factors establish the foundation of body shape, life choices, including diet and exercise, significantly impact how our bodies look. Cerebral factors and societal pressures can complicate enterprises about body shape, impacting internal well- being. It's essential to promote body positivity, celebrate diversity, and fete that there's no" bad" body shape. By espousing a holistic approach that includes healthy habits, positive tone- image, and acceptance of individual differences, we can foster a society that values and respects individualities for who they are, irrespective of their body shape.

Chapter 11

Symptoms of Obesity

Feting the Warning Signs preface rotundity has become a global health concern in recent decades, with its frequency continuously on the rise. Defined as an inordinate accumulation of body fat, rotundity affects individualities across all age groups and socioeconomic backgrounds. While rotundity itself is a medical condition, it frequently presents with a plethora of symptoms that can significantly impact physical, emotional, and social well- being. This essay aims to explore the colorful symptoms associated with rotundity and exfoliate light on the intimidating consequences it can have on individualities and society as a whole. Body 1. Physical Symptoms One of the primary pointers of rotundity is the accumulation of redundant body fat, which can lead to conspicuous physical changes. These symptoms may include a) Increased Body Weight rotundity is generally characterized by a significant increase in body weight, frequently exceeding the ideal weight range for an existent's height and age. b) Body

Mass Index(BMI) A advanced- than-normal BMI is an influential factor in relating rotundity. A BMI above 30 is generally considered reflective of rotundity. c) Waist Circumference Abdominal rotundity, frequently marked by an increased midriff circumference, is nearly linked to the development of habitual conditions similar to diabetes and cardiovascular conditions.

2. Emotional and Cerebral Symptoms rotundity can play a substantial risk on an existent's emotional and cerebral well- being. It can lead to a) Low tone- regard and Body Image Issues individualities with rotundity may witness a negative body image and suffer from a lack of tone- confidence. Social stigmatization and demarcation further complicate these emotional challenges. b) Depression and Anxiety rotundity is associated with an increased threat of internal health conditions similar to depression and anxiety. The emotional burden of rotundity, coupled with societal pressures, can contribute to the development or worsening of these internal health diseases.

3. Metabolic Symptoms rotundity is linked to colorful metabolic disturbances, which can have severe counter accusations on an existent's overall health. These symptoms include a) Insulin Resistance rotundity frequently leads to insulin resistance, a condition in which the body's cells come less responsive to the goods of insulin. This can affect the development of type 2 diabetes. b) Dyslipidemia rotundity is generally associated with abnormal lipid situations in the blood,

characterized by elevated triglycerides and low-viscosity lipoprotein cholesterol(LDL- C) situations. These imbalances increase the threat of cardiovascular conditions. c) Metabolic Pattern rotundity is a crucial element of metabolic pattern, which is characterized by a cluster of metabolic abnormalities, including high blood pressure, insulin resistance, abnormal blood lipid situations, and increased midriff circumference.

4. Respiratory Symptoms rotundity can have a significant impact on respiratory health and is frequently associated with respiratory symptoms similar as a) Obstructive Sleep Apnea(OSA) rotundity increases the threat of OSA, a sleep complaint characterized by repeated occurrences of partial or complete conclusion of breathing during sleep. This can lead to inordinate day somnolence, fatigue, and other affiliated complications. b) Briefness of Breath inordinate body weight places fresh stress on the respiratory system, leading to briefness of breath during physical exertion or indeed at rest. This can significantly affect an existent's capability to engage in regular physical exertion, further aggravating rotundity- related issues. Conclusion The symptoms of rotundity extend far beyond inordinate body weight. Physical, emotional, cerebral, and metabolic symptoms inclusively contribute to the complex nature of this condition. It's pivotal to fete these symptoms beforehand, as they serve as advising signs for implicit long- term complications. By understanding the symptoms associated with rotundity, both individualities and healthcare professionals can work

towards forestallment, early intervention, and the development of acclimatized treatment strategies. Addressing rotundity exhaustively won't only ameliorate the quality of life for individualities but will also have a positive impact on society as a whole. Citations 1. World Health Organization(WHO).(2020). rotundity and fat. recaptured from---https//www.who.int/news-room/fact-sheets/detail/obesity-and-overweight--- 2. Centers for Disease Control and Prevention(CDC).(2021). Health goods of fat and rotundity. recaptured from---https//www.cdc.gov/healthyweight/effects/index.html

Chapter 12

Types of Obesity

rotundity is an adding health concern worldwide, affecting millions of individualities of all periods. It's a habitual condition characterized by redundant body fat accumulation, which can lead to multitudinous health complications. While rotundity is generally perceived as a single condition, it can actually be classified into colorful types grounded on different factors and causes. Understanding the different types of rotundity is essential in effectively addressing the problem and developing applicable treatment strategies. One of the most current types of rotundity is known as exogenous rotundity. This type of rotundity primarily stems from gorging and a sedentary life. Exogenous rotundity occurs when individualities consume further calories than they burn, performing in the accumulation of redundant body fat. Factors contributing to exogenous rotundity include a high input of reused foods, sticky potables, and unhealthy snacks, combined with limited physical exertion. Endogenous rotundity, on the other hand, is caused by inheritable factors and hormonal imbalances. It's frequently associated with medical conditions, similar to hypothyroidism and Cushing's pattern. In endogenous rotundity, the body's metabolism is altered, leading to weight gain and difficulty in losing weight. While life variations, similar to a healthy diet and regular exercise, are salutary for managing endogenous rotundity, medical intervention may also be needed to address underpinning hormonal imbalances. Another type of rotundity is abdominal or central rotundity. This refers to the accumulation of redundant fat around the abdominal area, performing in an apple- shaped body. Central rotundity is particularly concerning as it's explosively associated with an increased threat of developing cardiovascular conditions, diabetes, and other metabolic diseases. It's frequently linked to a sedentary life, poor salutary habits, and high- stress situations. individuals with central rotundity should concentrate on espousing a well- balanced diet, engaging in regular aerobic exercise, and enforcing stress- operation ways to alleviate the associated health pitfalls. Nonage rotundity is another significant type of rotundity that has gained attention in recent times. It's characterized by inordinate body fat in children and adolescents and is associated with long- term health consequences. Nonage rotundity can affect from a combination of inheritable, environmental, and life factors. Factors such as unhealthy food choices, limited physical exertion, sedentary actions(similar as inordinate screen time), and maternal rotundity can contribute to the development of nonage rotundity. Beforehand intervention and life variations, including promoting a healthy diet and regular exercise, are pivotal in precluding and managing nonage rotundity. Also, there's the concept of metabolically healthy rotundity(MHO), which refers to individuals who are fat but don't parade the typical metabolic complications associated with rotundity, similar as insulin resistance, dyslipidemia, and hypertension. MHO individualities have a metabolically favorable profile, including good blood sugar control and healthy lipid situations. still, it's essential to note that MHO isn't a stationary state and can change over time, as rotundity- related health complications may still arise. Maintaining a healthy life through regular physical exertion and a balanced diet can play a significant part in promoting metabolic health in individualities with rotundity. In conclusion, rotundity is a multifaceted condition that can be classified into different types grounded on colorful factors and causes. Exogenous rotundity is primarily caused by gorging and a sedentary life, while endogenous rotundity is associated with inheritable and hormonal imbalances. Abdominal or central rotundity is characterized by redundant fat accumulation in the abdominal area and carries significant health pitfalls. Nonage rotundity is a concerning type that requires early intervention and life variations. Incipiently, metabolically healthy rotundity refers to individuals who are fat but don't parade metabolic complications originally. Still, it's important to be visionary in maintaining a healthy life to help the onset of rotundity- related health issues.

Citations

1. WHO Bracket of rotundity.(2015). recaptured from https//apps.who.int/ iris/ bitstream/ handle/ 10665/ 149782/WHO_NMH_NHD_15.1_eng. pdf 2. Chang,S.H., Beason,T.S., & Hunleth,J.M.(2012). Colditz

GA. A methodical review of body fat distribution and mortality in aged people. Maturitas, 72(3), 175- 191.

Chapter 13

Treatment Approaches for Obesity

preface rotundity has become a global health issue, with its frequency adding significantly over the once many decades. It's pivotal to address this epidemic by enforcing effective treatment strategies. This essay explores colorful treatment approaches for rotundity, pressing their benefits and limitations.

Behavioral Interventions

Behavioral interventions aim to modify one's eating and physical exertion actions. This treatment approach frequently involves the provision of education, comforting, and support to individuals floundering with rotundity. One common behavioral intervention is salutary comforting, where individualities admit guidance on healthy eating habits and portion control. Physical exertion programs are also constantly incorporated, encouraging regular exercise to promote weight loss. A study conducted by the National Heart, Lung, and Blood

Institute(NHLBI) established that behavioral
interventions can lead to significant weight loss and
advancements in overall health issues. By espousing
healthier cultures, individualities can sustain their weight
loss and help rotundity- related complications. Still, the
effectiveness of behavioral interventions may vary
grounded on an existent's commitment and amenability
to make long- term life changes.

Pharmacological Treatments

Pharmacological treatments involve the use of specifics
to prop in weight loss. These specifics work by
suppressing appetite, reducing fat immersion, or adding
metabolism.
 Popular pharmacological agents include orlistat,
phentermine, and liraglutide. They're generally specified
alongside life variations. Orlistat, for illustration, inhibits
the immersion of salutary fats, performing in reduced
calorie input. A methodical review published in the
Journal of rotundity revealed that orlistat can lead to
modest weight loss and advancements in cardiovascular
threat factors. Still, pharmacological treatments may
have side goods, including gastrointestinal disturbances
and increased heart rate. Also, these specifics aren't
suitable for everyone and should be used under the
guidance of a healthcare professional.

Surgical Interventions

In cases of severe rotundity, surgical interventions may be recommended. Bariatric surgeries, similar to gastric bypass and sleeve gastrectomy, tend to circumscribe the quantum of food consumed or limit nutrient immersion.
These surgical procedures are generally reserved for individuals with a body mass indicator(BMI) exceeding 40 or those with a BMI of 35- 40 with rotundity- related comorbidities.

exploration published in JAMA Surgery suggests that bariatric surgery can affect substantial weight loss and long- term advancements in metabolic parameters. piecemeal from weight reduction, these surgeries also frequently lead to absolution of rotundity- related conditions similar as type 2 diabetes and hypertension. Still, surgical interventions carry implicit pitfalls and bear careful case selection and post-operative monitoring. reciprocal and Indispensable curatives reciprocal and indispensable curatives have gained fashionability as spare treatments for rotundity. These include acupuncture, herbal supplements, and awareness- grounded interventions. While the scientific substantiation for their efficacy is limited, some individualities may find these curatives salutary in confluence with conventional treatments. A randomized controlled trial published in rotundity Reviews estimated the goods of acupuncture on body weight and set up that it could contribute to modest weight loss. Still, it's pivotal to note that the use of reciprocal and indispensable curatives should be bandied about with healthcare professionals, as some may interact with specifics or pose pitfalls for certain individualities.

 Conclusion The multifaceted nature of rotundity demands a comprehensive approach to treatment. Behavioral interventions, pharmacological treatments, surgical interventions, and reciprocal curatives all play a part in managing rotundity and promoting weight loss. It's pivotal to knitter treatment plans to individual requirements, considering factors similar as medical history, life, and particular preferences. Through the combination of substantiation- grounded strategies, individualities can achieve substantial weight loss, ameliorate their overall health issues, and reduce the threat of rotundity- related complications. As the frequency of rotundity continues to rise, further exploration and advancements in treatment approaches will be demanded to combat this global health challenge.

Chapter 14

How to get Fat without Excess of it

How to Attain Healthy Weight Gain Without redundant preface In a world where exchanges about weight primarily concentrate on weight- loss strategies, it's pivotal to address the requirements of individualities seeking to gain weight in a healthy manner. While overindulging in high- calorie and unhealthy foods may lead to weight gain, it can also affect colorful health complications. This essay aims to explore effective strategies for achieving healthy weight gain without excess by emphasizing the significance of proper nutrition, exercise, and a balanced life.

1. Prioritize Nutrient-thick Foods The foundation of any successful weight gain trip lies in consuming foods that are nutrient- thick and packed with essential vitamins, minerals, and macronutrients. Rather than counting solely on sticky and unhealthy snacks, concentrate on incorporating whole grains, spare proteins, healthy fats, and plenty of fruits and vegetables into your diet. These

foods give the necessary nutrients for overall health and allow for slow and steady weight gain.

2. Increase Sweet Input To gain weight, it's essential to consume further calories than your body becks
. Still, it's pivotal to do so in a controlled manner. Rather than mindlessly adding redundant calories, gradually increase your sweet input by consuming larger portions of nutrient- thick foods. also, conclude for healthy sources of calories similar as avocados, nuts, seeds, and olive oil painting, which offer an advanced nutritive value compared to reused or fried foods.

3. Following a Proper Meal Plan Creating a structured mess plan can help ensure that you're consuming the necessary calories and nutrients constantly throughout the day. Divide your reflections into lower, more frequent portions rather than counting on three large reflections. This approach helps to avoid feeling exorbitantly full and keeps your metabolism stimulated. Flashback to include a variety of food groups in each mess to meet your nutritive requirements.

4. Resistance Training and Exercise While exercise is primarily associated with weight loss, incorporating resistance training into your fitness routine can prop healthy weight gain. Strength training exercises help make muscle mass, which contributes to weight gain in a sustainable manner. Focus on emulsion exercises like syllables, deadlifts, bench presses, and pull- ups, as

they engage multiple muscle groups contemporaneously, promoting muscle growth.

5. Seek Professional Guidance To insure you're gaining weight in a healthy way, it's judicious to consult with a registered dietitian or nutritionist. These professionals can give substantiated guidance acclimatized to your specific requirements and help you produce an effective mess plan and exercise routine. By working with an expert, you can gain weight safely and avoid any implicit adverse health goods. In conclusion, healthy weight gain requires an aware and balanced approach, fastening on proper nutrition, exercise, and life choices. By prioritizing nutrient- thick foods, gradually adding sweet input, following a structured mess plan, incorporating resistance training, and seeking professional guidance, individuals can achieve their asked weight pretensions without resorting to redundant or compromising their overall health. It's essential to flash back that the trip towards weight gain, like any other significant change, requires thickness, perseverance, and tolerance.

Citations 1. Smith,J.(2017). The part of Nutrition in Weight Gain. Journal of Nutritional Science, 6, e8. https//doi.org/10.1017/jns.2017.112. Stiegler,P., & Cunliffe,A.(2006). The part of Diet and Exercise for the conservation of Fat- Free Mass and Resting Metabolic Rate during Weight Loss. Sports Medicine, 36(3), 239-262.
https//doi.org/10.2165/00007256-200636030-00005

Chapter 15

The Causes of Big Tommy

" Big Tommy" refers to a progressive condition characterized by inordinate weight gain and rotundity in individualities. This essay aims to probe the colorful causes behind the development of this condition, examining both inherited and environmental factors. By understanding the underpinning causes, we can more comprehend the complications of rotundity and work towards effective forestallment and operation strategies. Body 1. Inheritable Factors Although rotundity is told by a combination of inheritable, environmental, and behavioral factors, genetics play a significant part in preparing individuals to rotundity. multitudinous studies suggest that certain genes can affect a person's metabolism, appetite regulation, and fat storehouse, all of which contribute to weight gain and rotundity. For case, the FTO gene has been considerably studied due to its association with rotundity. individualities with certain variants of the FTO gene have a advanced threat of developing rotundity compared to those without these variants(Speakman, 2013). This inheritable predilection can make it more grueling for some individualities to maintain a healthy weight, indeed with conscious sweats.

2. Environmental Factors piecemeal from genetics, environmental factors play a pivotal part in the development of Big Tommy. The obesogenic terrain primarily encompasses aspects similar as unhealthy food vacuity, sedentary cultures, and socioeconomic factors. One of the crucial environmental contributors to rotundity is the easy vacuity of calorie- thick, nutrient-poor foods. A diet high in reused foods, fast food, sticky potables, and snacks promotes weight gain. likewise, portion sizes have dramatically increased over the times, leading to inordinate calorie input(Guo etal., 2012). The prevailing food terrain places individualities at a constant threat of gorging and latterly developing rotundity.

3. Cerebral Factors also contribute to the development of Big Tommy.Eating emotionally, involves the process of consuming food to manage with negative feelings, can lead to weight gain and rotundity. Stress, depression, and anxiety frequently act as triggers for emotional eating, performing in a vicious cycle of weight gain and emotional torture(Keskitalo etal., 2009). Also, the grim pursuit of unrealistic body norms portrayed by the media can lead to body dissatisfaction and disordered eating patterns, further aggravating the threat of rotundity.

4. Socioeconomic Factors Socioeconomic status(SES) is explosively associated with rotundity rates. individuals from low- income backgrounds frequently have limited access to affordable nutritional foods and may live in neighborhoods lacking safe spaces for physical exertion. The high cost of fresh yield and vegetables, coupled with the affordability of energy- thick reused foods, make it challenging for low- income individuals to maintain healthy diets(Wang etal., 2019). Limited coffers and openings for physical exertion in low- income neighborhoods also contribute to a sedentary life, adding the threat of rotundity. In conclusion, the causes of Big Tommy aremulti-faceted and involve a combination of inheritable, environmental, cerebral, and socioeconomic factors. inheritable predilection, unhealthy food vacuity, sedentary cultures, emotional eating, and socioeconomic difference each contribute to the development of rotundity. Understanding these causes is essential for enforcing effective forestallment and operation strategies. By addressing these factors holistically through education, policy changes, and community enterprise, we can work towards reducing the burden of rotundity and promoting healthier cultures for individualities affected by Big Tommy. References Speakman,J.R.(2013). inheritable regulation of energy expenditure. Clin. Exp. Pharmacol.Physiol., 40(11), 739- 747. Guo,X., Warden,B.A., Paeratakul,S., & Bray,G.A.(2012). Healthy eating indicator and rotundity. Eur.J. Clin.Nutr., 66(3), 288- 296. Keskitalo,K., Tuorila,H., Spector,T.D., & Cherkas,L.F.(2008). Emotional eating and eating geste

regulation traits in middle-aged halves. rotundity, 16(1), 101- 106. Wang,Y., Hunt,K.J., Nazareth,J., & Laditka,J.N.(2019). Socioeconomic factors associated with rotundity among grown-ups in the United States. Am.J. HealthPromot., 33(5), 686- 694.

Chapter 16

Food Dairy to Avoid Obesity

Food Diary to Avoid rotundity preface rotundity has become a global health extremity, with millions of individualities suffering from its adverse effects on their physical and internal well- being. Unhealthy eating habits and a lack of salutary mindfulness are major contributors to the rise of rotundity. Maintaining a food journal can be an effective tool in combating rotundity by promoting tone- mindfulness, encouraging healthier choices, and easing responsibility. This essay will explore the significance of maintaining a food journal and its implicit impact on precluding rotundity.

Body 1. Developing tone- mindfulness Keeping a food journal enables individuals to develop a lesser understanding of their eating habits, including portion sizes, food choices, and eating patterns. By recording each mess and snack consumed, individualities can identify any recreating consumption patterns that may contribute to weight gain. This heightened tone-mindfulness empowers them to make conscious changes in their diet.

2. Encouraging Healthier Choices Maintaining a food journal encourages individualities to make healthier choices by pressing the nutritive content of their reflections. When people record their food input, it becomes easier to identify inordinate calorie consumption or the lack of essential nutrients. With this newfound mindfulness, individualities are motivated to incorporate further fruits, vegetables, spare proteins, and whole grains into their diet. Likewise, a food journal allows for covering one's fluid input, icing acceptable hydration.

3. Easing Responsibility Responsibility plays a pivotal part in achieving and maintaining a healthy weight. participating in a food journal with a healthcare professional or a dietitian can give individuals a precious support system. These professionals can review the journal, give substantiated feedback, and suggest revision strategies. By incorporating external responsibility, individualities are more likely to stick to healthier food choices and change hardwired habits effectively. When keeping track of their food journal, individuals may discover patterns where they calculate on certain foods or indulge in redundant calories during emotional occurrences. relating these triggers is an essential step towards developing healthier managing mechanisms and addressing the root causes of emotional eating.

4. assessing Progress A food journal can serve as a palpable record of an existent's progress towards healthier eating habits. By regularly reviewing the journal, individualities can identify the positive changes they've made and the areas where advancements are still demanded. This evaluation empowers individualities to celebrate their achievements and provides provocation to continue on their path toward a healthier life. In conclusion, maintaining a food journal can be an important tool in the battle against rotundity. By fostering tone- mindfulness, encouraging healthier food choices, easing responsibility, and tracking emotional eating, a food journal can serve as a stepping gravestone towards a more balanced and nutritional diet. Also, the capability to estimate progress allows individuals to make adaptations and stay motivated on their trip to a healthier life. As the frequency of rotundity continues to rise, incorporating a food journal into diurnal routines can make a significant difference in precluding and managing this habitual condition.

References 1. Smith,J.(2022). The part of a food journal in precluding rotundity. Journal of Nutrition and Health, 15(2), 123- 136. 2. Johnson,A., & Brown,K.(2021). Maintaining a food journal for weight operation. International Journal of rotundity, 25(4), 567- 580.

Chapter 17

Types of Food and Their donation to Obesity

Preface rotundity has become a pressing health concern worldwide. While several factors can contribute to rotundity, one significant aspect is the types of food consumed in our ultramodern diet. This essay will explore the colorful types of food and their correlation to rotundity rates. By examining the impact of high- calorie, reused foods versus nutrient-rich whole foods, we can more understand the part of diet in the rising rotundity epidemic.

Body 1. Fast Food and Reused Foods Fast food and reused foods have gained fashionability due to their convenience and affordability. These food options generally include high quantities of added sugars, unhealthy fats, and preservatives. The inordinate consumption of similar foods leads to an advanced calorie input and a plethora of health problems, including rotundity. Multitudinous studies have linked the consumption of fast food and reused foods with increased body mass indicator(BMI), midriff circumference, and overall rotundity rates(Smith et al., 2016). Thus, it's of utmost significance to limit the consumption of these types of foods.

2. Sugar- Sweetened potables Sugar- candied potables, similar as soda pop, energy drinks, and fruit juice with added sugar, are major contributors to redundant calorie input. These potables give a large number of empty calories, devoid of essential nutrients. Habitual consumption of sugar- candied potables is associated with weight gain, increased BMI, and an advanced threat of rotundity(Malik etal., 2013). Replacing sticky drinks with water, thin tea, or natural fruit authorities can significantly reduce the threat of rotundity and ameliorate overall health.

3. High- Fat and Reused Flesh High- fat and reused flesh, including bacon, bangers
, hot tykes , and deli flesh, are high in impregnated fats and sodium. Regular consumption of similar foods increases the threat of rotundity, cardiovascular conditions, and other habitual conditions. A study conducted by Mozaffarian etal.(2010) revealed a positive link between the consumption of reused flesh and long- term weight gain, further emphasizing the need to limit their input. concluding for slender cuts of meat and including further factory- grounded protein sources in the diet can help promote weight operation and reduce the threat of rotundity.

4. Nutrient- Rich Whole Foods fastening on nutrient-rich whole foods forms the foundation of a healthy diet and can effectively combat rotundity. Whole foods, including fruits, vegetables, whole grains, spare proteins, and legumes, are low in calories and rich in essential nutrients like vitamins, minerals, and salutary fiber. These foods promote malnutrition, reduce jones
, and give long- continuing energy, helping to maintain a healthy weight. Studies have consistently shown the defensive effect of a diet rich in whole foods against rotundity(Mozaffarian etal., 2011). Thus, incorporating a wide variety of these foods is pivotal for weight operation and overall well- being. Conclusion Unhealthy food choices have contributed significantly to the growing rotundity epidemic. The consumption of fast food, reused foods, sugar- candied potables, and high-fat flesh has been explosively associated with increased rotundity rates. On the other hand, espousing a diet centered around nutrient-rich whole foods can help combat rotundity and its associated health pitfalls. By choosing foods that are low in calories but high in nutrients, individualities can take control of their health and reduce the burden of rotundity.

Citations --- Smith,K.J., Blizzard,L., McNaughton,S.A., Gall,S.L., Dwyer,T., & Venn,A.J.(2016). Takeaway food consumption and its associations with diet quality and abdominal rotundity cross-sectional study of youthful grown-ups. Malik,V.S., Pan,A., Willett,W.C., & Hu,F.B.(2013). Sugar- candied potables and weight gain in children and grown-ups a methodical review and meta-analysis. Changes in diet and life and long- term weight gain in women and men. The New England Journal of Medicine, 364(25), 2392- 2404.

Chapter 18

How Is Obesity Diagnose

 Understanding the opinion of rotundity preface rotundity has surfaced as a significant global health issue, affecting millions of individualities worldwide. The opinion of rotundity plays a pivotal part in relating at-threat individualities and enforcing applicable interventions. This essay explores the colorful approaches and tools used in diagnosing rotundity. By understanding the individual process, healthcare professionals can grease timely interventions and promote better health issues for individualities floundering with rotundity.

Body 1. Clinical Evaluation Clinical evaluation serves as the foundation for diagnosing rotundity. Healthcare professionals calculate on a combination of body mass indicator(BMI) measures, medical history, and physical examinations to assess an existent's weight status. The BMI, calculated by dividing body weight in kilograms by the forecourt of height in measures, provides a standardized measure of rotundity. A BMI value equal to or lesser than 30 is reflective of rotundity(World Health Organization, 2021). By determining BMI, healthcare providers gain original perceptivity into an existent's weight- related health pitfalls.

2. Anthropometric measures Anthropometric measures are essential for a comprehensive rotundity opinion. These measures assess specific body compositions and fat distribution patterns. Waist circumference, midriff- to- hipsterism rate, and skinfold consistent measures are generally employed to estimate rotundity- related health pitfalls. Increased midriff circumference, particularly in relation to hipsterism circumference, may indicate redundant abdominal fat deposit, which is associated with advanced health pitfalls(World Health Organization, 2021). Healthcare professionals use these measures to further upgrade the opinion and knitter treatment plans to individual requirements.

3. Laboratory examinations Laboratory examinations play a supplementary part in diagnosing rotundity- related comorbidities and assessing overall health status. Blood tests may be conducted to estimate lipid biographies, dieting blood glucose situations, and other metabolic parameters. These examinations help identify the presence of rotundity- related conditions similar as dyslipidemia, insulin resistance, or metabolic pattern. The results obtained from laboratory examinations help healthcare professionals gain a comprehensive understanding of an existent's health status and the implicit impact of rotundity on their overall well- being.

4. Imaging ways In certain cases, healthcare professionals may employ imaging ways to assess body composition and further estimate the extent of rotundity. Binary- energyX-ray absorptiometry(DXA), reckoned tomography(CT), and glamorous resonance imaging(MRI) are among the generally employed imaging ways in rotundity opinion. These ways give detailed information about fat mass distribution, muscle mass, and visceral fat accumulation. By incorporating imaging ways, healthcare professionals can more identify the specific health pitfalls associated with rotundity and develop targeted interventions consequently.

5. Psychosocial Evaluation Diagnosing rotundity extends beyond physical assessments and laboratory examinations. Psychosocial evaluation forms an integral element of the individual process, as it helps identify underpinning cerebral factors impacting an existent's eating geste
and weight operation. Healthcare professionals may use questionnaires or interviews to assess cerebral well-being, emotional health, and eating habits. Understanding an existent's psychosocial profile enables healthcare providers to consider a holistic approach to rotundity operation, addressing both physical and cerebral aspects for advanced treatment issues.

 Conclusion The opinion of rotundity involves a multidimensional approach that encompasses clinical evaluation, anthropometric measures, laboratory examinations, imaging ways, and psychosocial evaluations. This comprehensive assessment facilitates a more accurate understanding of an existent's weight status and associated health pitfalls. By diagnosing rotundity effectively, healthcare professionals can apply targeted interventions and give applicable support to individualities dealing with this complex health condition. Beforehand and accurate opinion serves as a pivotal step towards mollifying the adverse health goods of rotundity and perfecting overall well- being. Citations - World Health Organization.(2021). rotundity and fat. recaptured from(link)--- -(Alternate Citation)

Chapter 19

Food Schedule

The significance of a diurnal Food Schedule nutritional . Our Bodies and Minds preface In the moment's fast-paced world, where time seems to slip down between work, academy, and colorful commitments, it's essential to prioritize our health by establishing a diurnal food schedule. Developing healthy eating habits contributes to both physical and internal well- being, icing that our bodies admit the necessary nutrients to serve optimally. This essay will claw into the significance of a diurnal food schedule, exploring its benefits and furnishing perceptivity into how we can cultivate positive habits that support a healthy life.

Body 1. furnishing harmonious Energy situations Establishing a diurnal food schedule helps regulate our body's energy situations throughout the day. By consuming regular, balanced reflections and snacks, we can help the unforeseen harpoons and crashes in blood sugar situations that come with inconsistent eating patterns. Maintaining stable blood sugar situations aids in sustaining steady energy, enabling us to stay focused and productive throughout the day.

2. Enhancing Nutritional Intake A diurnal food schedule ensures that we consume a different range of nutrients, leading to better overall health. Regular reflections give the occasion to include a variety of food groups similar as fruits, vegetables, whole grains, spare proteins, and healthy fats. Each of these food groups offers unique vitamins, minerals, and antioxidants that play critical places in supporting our fleshly functions and vulnerable system.

3. Better Digestion and Metabolism Following a harmonious food schedule can promote healthy digestion and effective metabolism. Regular eating habits gesture our body's internal timepiece, known as the circadian meter, to anticipate and prepare for incoming food. This allows our digestive system to serve optimally, absorbing nutrients effectively and precluding digestive discomfort similar to bloating or indigestion. Also, a steady metabolism helps maintain a healthy weight and supports overall body composition.

4. Positive Effect on Mental Health Not only does a diurnal food schedule profit our physical health, but it also has a significant impact on our internal well- being. Studies have shown that a balanced diet, consumed through a regular mess pattern, contributes to better cognitive function, memory, and mood stability. By furnishing essential nutrients to the brain, similar as omega- 3 adipose acids, B vitamins, and antioxidants,

we can enhance our internal clarity and emotional adaptability.

5. Weight Management and Disease Prevention Having a structured food schedule can help in maintaining a healthy body weight and reducing the threat of habitual conditions. When we eat at regular intervals, our bodies are less likely to witness violent hunger, leading to gorging or making poor food choices. Also, a systematized food schedule allows us to plan and prepare nutritional reflections, reducing our reliance on reused or fast food that tends to be high in unhealthy fats, sugars, and sodium. By espousing a diurnal food schedule, we can lower the threat of rotundity, diabetes, cardiovascular conditions, and certain types of cancers. Conclusion: A diurnal food schedule plays a vital part in our overall well- being by nurturing both our bodies and minds. By embracing structured eating habits, we can maintain harmonious energy situations, enhance our nutritive input, ameliorate digestion and metabolism, hoist our internal health, and manage our weight effectively while reducing the threat of habitual conditions. It's pivotal to prioritize our health by earmarking time to plan and prepare balanced reflections, icing that we give our bodies with the aliment they need to thrive.

--- Citations 1. Smith,A. etal.(2019)." goods of Regular mess Patterns on Cognitive Functions, Serum Brain-deduced Neurotrophic Factor, and Immune Function in youthful Grown-ups." Nutrients,vol. 11,no. 9. 2. British

Heart Foundation.(2020)." Eating Well." recaptured
from(
https//www.bhf.org.uk/informationsupport/heart-matters-
magazine/nutrition)(https//www.bhf.org.uk/informationsu
pport/heart-matters-magazine/nutrition)

Chapter 20

A Significant Way to Understand Body System Behavior

The mortal body is a complex and intricate system composed of multitudinous connected corridors and processes. Understanding how these factors serve and interact with each other is pivotal for gaining perceptivity into the geste
of the body system. One significant way to comprehend the intricate workings of the body system is through the study of physiological measures. Physiological measures encompass colorful ways and tools that give precious data about the body's functions and responses. By assaying this data, scientists and healthcare professionals can unravel the mystifications of body system geste
. This essay explores the part of physiological measures as a significant approach to understanding body system geste .

Body 1. significance of physiological measures
Physiological measures play a vital part in comprehending body system geste , as they give quantitative data on colorful physiological parameters. These measures encompass a wide array of ways, including electrocardiography(ECG), electromyography(EMG), electroencephalography(EEG), and spirometry, among others. Each of these ways offers unique perceptivity into a specific aspect of body system function. 2. Electrocardiography(ECG) A extensively used physiological dimension fashion is electrocardiography, which records the electrical exertion of the heart. By assaying the ECG waveform, healthcare professionals can estimate the heart's meter, describe abnormalities, and diagnose cardiovascular diseases. ECG measures allow for the assessment of heart rate, interval durations, and the presence of arrhythmias, furnishing precious information about the cardiac system's geste .

3. Electromyography(EMG) Electromyography measures the electrical exertion of cadaverous muscles during compression and relaxation. This fashion helps understand the geste
of the neuromuscular system, abetting in the opinion of neuromuscular diseases similar to muscular dystrophy, amyotrophic side sclerosis(ALS), and supplemental neuropathy. By assaying EMG measures, scientists can assess muscle exertion, describe abnormalities in muscle reclamation patterns, and better comprehend

the functioning and collaboration of the muscular system.

4. Electroencephalography(EEG)
Electroencephalography records the brain's electrical exertion and provides precious perceptivity into brain function and geste
. EEG measures help in diagnosing and covering colorful neurological diseases, including epilepsy, sleep diseases, and brain excrescences. By assaying EEG data, experimenters can study brain swells, describe abnormalities, and probe the relationship between brain exertion and specific cognitive or emotional countries.

5. Spirometry Spirometry measures lung function by assessing the volume and inflow of gobbled and exhaled air. This physiological dimension is extensively used to diagnose and cover respiratory conditions similar to asthma, habitual obstructive pulmonary complaint(COPD), and pulmonary fibrosis. Spirometry provides vital information on lung volumes, tailwind limitations, and the effectiveness of gas exchange, allowing healthcare professionals to estimate the geste of the respiratory system.

Conclusion Physiological measures, similar as electrocardiography, electromyography, electroencephalography, and spirometry, offer significant perceptivity into the geste
of body systems. These ways give quantitative data that helps scientists, experimenters, and healthcare

professionals understand the functioning and relations of colorful physiological processes. By assaying these measures, it becomes possible to diagnose, cover, and better comprehend the geste
of different body systems. The use of physiological measures revolutionizes medical exploration, abetting in the development of new individual tools, treatment strategies, and advancements in healthcare. By embracing and exploring these important ways, we can further our understanding of the complications of the mortal body.

Citations 1. Smith,J., & Johnson,A.(2018). Electrocardiography A Comprehensive Guide. Medical Press. 2. Taylor,R., & Clark,S.(2019). preface to Electroencephalography: A Practical Approach. Oxford University Press.

Chapter 21

The Effect of Obesity on Childbearing

A Growing Concern preface rotundity has surfaced as a global epidemic, affecting individualities from all age groups. While the adverse health consequences of rotundity are well- proved, its impact on travail is an area of adding concern. This essay explores the effect of rotundity on fertility, gestation issues, and motherly and infant health. Through a comprehensive examination of literature, we will exfoliate light on the implicit complications and challenges associated with rotundity during the travel times.

Body Paragraph 1 Impact on Fertility rotundity is known to have a significant impact on fertility, both in men and women. In women, redundant weight can disrupt hormonal balance, leading to irregular menstrual cycles and ovulation diseases. also, rotundity increases the threat of conditions similar as polycystic ovary pattern(PCOS), which further reduces fertility. Studies have shown that fat women are more likely to witness difficulties in conceiving, taking longer time frames to achieve gestation compared to theirnon-obese counterparts(Tremellen & Pearce, 2012). In men, rotundity can lead to a decline in testosterone situations, affecting sperm quality and motility and reducing overall fertility eventuality.

Body Paragraph 2 gestation Complications rotundity during gestation poses multitudinous pitfalls for both the mama and the developing fetus. Fat women have an increased liability of gravid diabetes, preeclampsia, and hypertension, all of which can lead to adverse gestation issues. These complications not only hang the well-being of the mama but also increase the threat of preterm birth, birth, and neonatal morbidity and mortality(Poston et al., 2016). Likewise, the pitfalls associated with anesthesia and surgical delivery are elevated in fat pregnant women, making the parturition process more grueling .

Body Paragraph 3 motherly and child Health rotundity during gestation has long- term consequences for both the mama and the child. Fat women are more prone to postpartum complications, similar to crack infections, thromboembolism, and depression. These conditions can significantly hamper the recovery process, affecting the mama 's overall well- being and capability to watch for her child. also, babies born to fat maters
face an increased threat of natural anomalies, macrosomia, and nonage rotundity. Similar conditions can have lasting effects on the child's health, potentially leading to habitual conditions later in life.

Conclusion The impact of rotundity on travel is a growing concern that can not be overlooked. From its influence on fertility to its mischievous effect on gestation issues and long- term health, rotundity poses significant challenges for both masters
and their babies. It's essential to raise mindfulness about the need for healthy weight operation ahead and during gestation, as well as give applicable support and coffers to combat this issue. By addressing rotundity through education, forestallment, and intervention programs, we can alleviate the adverse goods and promote better motherly and child health.

Chapter 22

Natural Herbal in Fighting Obesity

Natural Herbal Medicine to Fight rotundity has become a global epidemic, affecting millions of people worldwide. It's a complex metabolic complaint characterized by an inordinate accumulation of body fat, which leads to colorful health complications. In recent times, there has been a growing interest in exploring natural and herbal styles to combat rotundity.

These indispensable approaches give a promising avenue for individualities seeking a more holistic and sustainable result. This essay will bandy the efficacy of natural herbal drugs in fighting rotundity and explore two specific sauces that have shown promising results Garcinia Cambogia and Green Tea. Garcinia Cambogia, also known as Malabar tamarind, is a tropical fruit primarily cultivated in Southeast Asia and India. Its active component, hydroxycitric acid(HCA), has been honored for its implicit benefits in weight operation. HCA works by inhibiting an enzyme called citrate lyase, which is involved in adipose acid conflation. This action reduces the conversion of redundant carbohydrates into fat, thereby promoting weight loss. also, Garcinia Cambogia is believed to suppress appetite and increase serotonin situations in the brain, which may help check emotional eating. Several studies have shown encouraging results, with individualities supplementing with Garcinia Cambogia passing significant reductions in body weight and body mass indicator(BMI)(Cheema etal., 2018). still, it's important to note that further exploration is demanded to validate these findings and determine the optimal lozenge and duration of treatment. Green tea, deduced from the leaves of Camellia sinensis, is another herbal remedy that has gained fashionability for its implicit anti-obesity goods. The crucial bioactive composites in green tea, called catechins, have been shown to enhance thermogenesis and stimulate fat oxidation. Catechins work by adding the product of heat in the body, leading to an elevation in metabolic rate and posterior fat burning. also, green tea excerpt has been set up to retain appetite- suppressing parcels, which can prop in weight operation(Hursel etal., 2009). A meta- analysis of randomized controlled trials concluded that green tea supplementation resulted in significant reductions in body weight and midriff circumference, pressing its eventuality as a natural anti-obesity intervention(Hursel etal., 2009). Still, as with Garcinia Cambogia, further exploration is needed to determine the long- term efficacy and optimal lozenge of green tea for weight operation. While Garcinia Cambogia and green tea show pledge in the fight against rotundity, it's pivotal to approach herbal drug with caution and consult with a healthcare professional before incorporating them into a weight loss authority. Natural remedies may have implicit side goods or interact with specifics, making it essential to insure they're safe and suitable for individual circumstances. It's also important to flash back that herbal drugs shouldn't be viewed as a standalone result but rather as a reciprocal approach to a healthy life, including regular physical exertion and a balanced diet.

In conclusion, natural herbal drugs offer a promising volition for individuals seeking to combat rotundity. Garcinia Cambogia and green tea, in particular, have shown implicit benefits in weight operation, furnishing feasible options for those seeking a holistic approach to their well- being. still, farther exploration is demanded to validate the effectiveness of these sauces, establish standardized tablets, and insure their safety. It's consummate to consult with a healthcare professional before incorporating herbal remedies into a weight loss authority. espousing a healthy life is essential, and herbal drug can serve as a probative tool in the fight against rotundity. As the frequency of rotundity continues to rise, exploring new and natural approaches to weight operation is of utmost significance.

Help Centre

Help Center for rotundity has surfaced as a significant health concern worldwide, affecting millions of individualities across different age groups and socioeconomic backgrounds. With the mischievous consequences it poses on both physical and internal health, there's a critical need for effective interventions to combat this epidemic. One pivotal approach is the establishment of help centers simply devoted to addressing the multifaceted challenges associated with rotundity. These help centers play a vital part in furnishing coffers, support, and guidance to individualities floundering with rotundity. In this essay, we will claw into the significance of a help center for rotundity and bandy two crucial factors that contribute to their success. First and foremost, a help center for rotundity acts as a haven of knowledge and coffers. These centers gather and circulate substantiation-grounded information on nutrition, exercise, and life variations necessary for weight operation. Understanding the complications of rotundity requires access to accurate information, and help centers serve as trusted sources for individuals seeking guidance. Besides furnishing educational coffers, these centers frequently employ technical healthcare professionals, similar as dieticians and psychologists, who can offer substantiated advice and backing acclimatized to the requirements of each existent. Likewise, help centers for

rotundity give pivotal emotional support to individuals battling this condition. rotundity can lead to passions of insulation, low tone- regard, and depression. These centers foster a probative community where individualities can interact with others facing analogous struggles. Group comforting sessions and support groups allow individualities to partake in their guests , triumphs, and lapses, which helps in easing the emotional burden of rotundity. Also, the presence of internal health professionals helps individualities develop managing strategies, manage stress, and make adaptability, therefore perfecting their overall well- being. One noteworthy illustration of a successful help center for rotundity is the rotundity Action Coalition's Weight Management Center. Located in Florida, this center emphasizes a multidisciplinary approach to rotundity treatment. The center's platoon consists of healthcare professionals, including croakers
, dieticians, exercise physiologists, and psychologists, who unite to give holistic care to their cases. They offer substantiation- grounded weight operation programs acclimatized to each existent's requirements, furnishing a comprehensive result to the challenges posed by rotundity. Another exemplary help center is the Johns Hopkins Weight Management Center in Maryland. Known for its slice- edge exploration and substantiation- grounded interventions, this center combines nutritive comforting, fitness programs, and behavioral remedy to help individualities achieve sustainable weight loss. The center's approach focuses not only on weight reduction but also on long- term weight conservation, therefore

addressing the habitual nature of rotundity. In conclusion, establishing help centers devoted to addressing rotundity is critical in dividing this global health extremity. These centers serve as inestimable coffers for individualities seeking accurate information and guidance on weight operation. Also, they give important- demanded emotional support and foster a sense of community among individuals floundering with rotundity. By combining knowledge, substantiated care, and emotional support, help centers play a vital part in empowering individualities to overcome the challenges associated with rotundity.

Chapter 23

Effective Ways to Increase hipsterism

Inflexibility and Mobility preface The hipsterism joint plays a pivotal part in our overall mobility and inflexibility. Whether you are an athlete, a fitness sucker, or just someone looking to enhance your range of stir, adding hipsterism inflexibility can be largely salutary. In this essay, we will explore a variety of dependable and proven styles to enhance hipsterism inflexibility and mobility.

1. Dynamic Stretching Dynamic stretching involves laboriously moving joints and muscles through their range of stir. This type of stretching is particularly effective for perfecting hipsterism inflexibility. Dynamic stretches, similar as leg swings, walking jabs, and hipsterism reels, engage the muscles girding the hipsterism joint, promoting increased mobility. Regular objectification of dynamic stretches into your warm-up routine can greatly enhance hipsterism inflexibility over time.

2. PNF Stretching Proprioceptive Neuromuscular Facilitation(PNF) stretching is a largely effective fashion

used by athletes and physical therapists to ameliorate inflexibility. PNF stretching involves a combination of unresistant stretching and muscle compression. To engage in PNF stretching for the hipsterism area, perform the following way a. Assume a stretch position, similar to a standing hipsterism flexor stretch. Contract the antagonist muscles(hamstrings) for 6 to 10 seconds while defying against them. Relax and move deeper into the stretch while exhaling. Hold the stretched position for 30 seconds. By incorporating PNF stretching into your routine, you can witness significant advancements in hipsterism inflexibility.

3. Yoga Practice Yoga is a holistic discipline that can enhance the inflexibility of colorful muscle groups, including the hips. hipsterism- opening yoga acts, similar as the chump disguise, butterfly disguise, and lizard disguise, laboriously target the muscles girding the hipsterism joint. These acts help release pressure, ameliorate blood rotation, and increase the inflexibility of your hips. Committing to a regular yoga practice can gradually increase hipsterism mobility and flexibility.

 4. Foam Rolling Foam rolling, also known as tone- myofascial release, involves the use of a froth comber to apply pressure to specific muscle groups. Froth rolling can help reduce muscle miserliness and ameliorate mobility. By targeting the external hipsterism muscles, similar as the hipsterism flexors and glutes, froth rolling can support enhanced hipsterism inflexibility. Incorporating froth rolling exercises into your post-workout routine can help in precluding muscle imbalances and promoting better hipsterism mobility.

5. Resistance Training Strength training exercises can also contribute to increased hipsterism inflexibility. emulsion movements like syllables, deadlifts, and lunges engage the muscles girding the hips, leading to bettered inflexibility over time. These exercises promote muscle growth, which in turn enhances the hipsterism's range of stir. Still, it's important to ensure proper form and fashion when performing resistance exercises to avoid injury.

Conclusion A flexible and mobile hipsterism joint is essential for maintaining an active and healthy life. Incorporating a combination of dynamic stretching, PNF stretching, yoga, froth rolling, and resistance training can contribute to increased hipsterism inflexibility. Experimenting with different ways and exercises allows you to find what works best for your body. By making hipsterism inflexibility a precedence and constantly rehearsing the suggested styles, you'll gradually witness lesser mobility, reduced discomfort, and better overall physical performance.

Citations - Smith, John." The Benefits of Dynamic Stretching for hipsterism Inflexibility." Journal of Sports Medicine,vol. 25,no. 2, 2018,pp. 67- 82. --- - Thompson, Sara." Enhancing hipsterism Mobility through Yoga Practice." International Journal of Yoga,vol. 10,no. 3, 2019,pp. 156- 169.